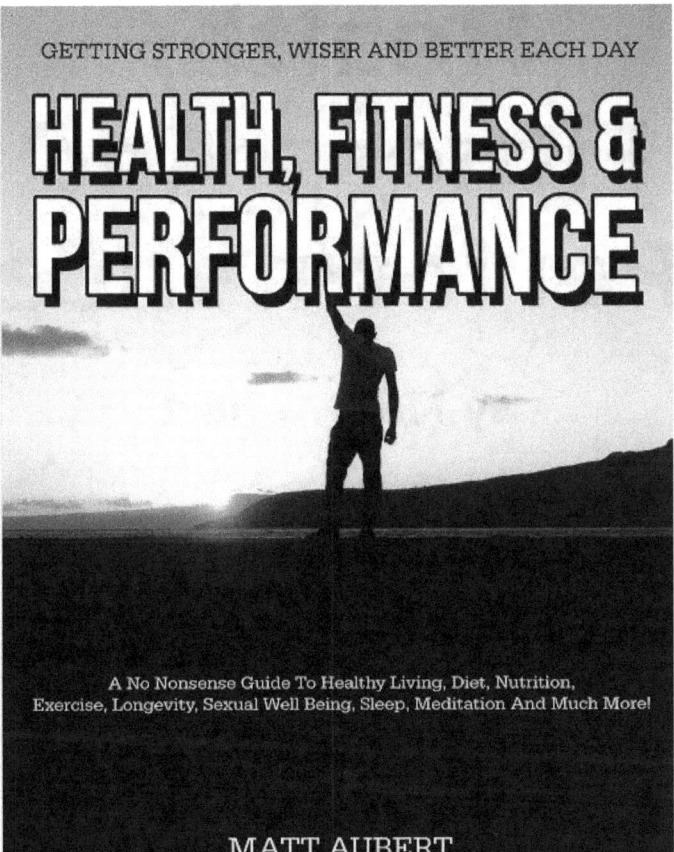

GETTING STRONGER, WISER AND BETTER EACH DAY

HEALTH, FITNESS & PERFORMANCE

A No Nonsense Guide To Healthy Living, Diet, Nutrition,
Exercise, Longevity, Sexual Well Being, Sleep, Meditation And Much More!

MATT AUBERT

Health, Fitness And Performance

By Matt Aubert

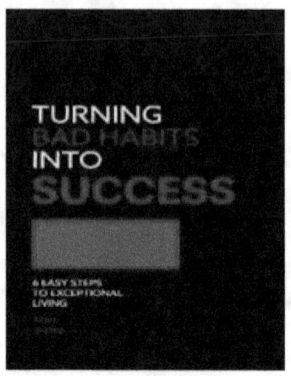

FREE DOWNLOAD

Sign up for the author's New Releases mailing list and get a free copy of the latest Turning Bad Habits into Success.

Click here to get started:
www.StartLiving.com

Table of Contents

I wrote "Health, Fitness and Performance" based on so many people hard at work and are really trying to get "ahead" in life with this health/exercise thing BUT are failing miserably. Not being harsh but those are called the facts.

I competed in bicycle freestyle contests growing up which helped me stay in shape. Upon graduating high school I joined the military and my physical fitness really started taking off. Every morning physical training took place with the troops and running a minimum of 2 miles daily!

After serving my country I also became a certified personal trainer at Bally Total Fitness in Atlanta, GA where I trained literally hundreds of people. Old, young, experienced or inexperienced, it didn't matter. My job was to help them achieve their fitness goals and that's exactly what I did.

Now my services were not free nor where they cheap. But honestly if I wasn't there to help some of them they might not have done anything!

My first workout with them was always free which gave them a chance to see what I could do for them. Sort of similar to test driving a car or trying on an outfit.

This is where I would find out if they had previous injuries or what medications they took which is typical with any training program. Finding this information out was critical and part of being a personal trainer. At the end of the session I would discuss prices for the different training packages which went upwards of $3,500 for 48 sessions.

Invariably they would many times say they didn't have the money or could not afford it at the time. But little did they know while I was questioning them that first hour before training them I was building my case. I would ask if they smoked, how many times they went out and had some drinks or just out to eat. While they were talking I was adding this stuff up!

Guess what? They DID have the money but it was going to other things such as cigarettes, eating out and drinking some adult beverages! Don't get me wrong we all need to enjoy life but not at the expense of $500-1000 a month!

As I was interviewing them about their physical goals I would interject a question here and there concerning their lifestyle which gave me insight on where their hard earn dollars were truly going. Funny thing was they didn't even realize how much they were spending on this stuff!

Once I explained their situation to them and put them into the context then they would say "Wow I never knew I spent that much money on this stuff". Next they would sign up and purchase training.

FACT: People underestimate restaurant meals by 700 calories

I've been a student of healthy living my entire life and I can tell you one thing for sure. If you do not seek out information and become a student of healthy living you will have difficulty with almost anything and everything you do in life.

Let's take for instance that you won a $1,000,000 which would be pretty awesome. Guess what, if you're not healthy enough then how can you enjoy the money and do anything with it? You see people never connect the two. But you'll hear them tell you what they would be doing IF they were to come in contact with that kind of money.

To be quite honest think about where people that are out of shape would wind up if they really won a million dollars. Their jobs are probably the only exercise they receive. So winning a million bucks would have them basically turn into a true couch potato since they don't have to work anymore. Counterproductive to say the least.

This could be their doom instead of their destiny!

Another thing people will tell you is they need to get in better shape. But do these folks really mean it? Probably not based on them not doing anything about it. Words alone have never gotten a person in shape. Ever.

Remember a body in motion stays in motion.

Do something different in the next 90 days than you did the last 90 days.

People take care of their yards, work, car, job, house and everything else but never their own bodies. Why is that?

You have to start somewhere and now is the best time. Don't wait another minute, another hour or day, make today your starting point to achieving the body you've always talked about and this will ensure your health will not suffer so that when you are older you don't look it or feel it!

Another point of interest I want to bring to the table.

Most people never read past the first chapter of any book they purchase. Another intriguing fact is only 1/3 of adults read a book after graduating school!

My point is to NOT be one of these statistics.

As you're reading make notes in the book, write down ideas you get as they come to you, and use this as a reference.

Don't rely on your memory because you will not remember. Don't read this once and move on. Read it again and again and I'll guarantee you that you will get something new from it every time.

I have ALWAYS gotten something new after reading a book again. As a matter of fact every time I listen to a CD or read a book again I have learned something new that I didn't catch the first or second or third time.

Once you understand how important living a healthy life truly is and actually apply these principles you will be much further ahead of the pack.

Use what I've created as a reference and continue to learn new ideas and principles. Become a student in this life long journey of being healthy and never stop growing!

I wish you much success and will see you at the top my friend!

Unfortunately I do not know you. I'm not familiar with your dreams or your problems. Fortunately that doesn't matter because what I'm about to tell you is universal and works either way.

People always come up to me and wonder what the secret is to healthy living. My answer is always the same and that's you must start with your own thought process.

What do I mean by this? I mean WHY do you want to increase your health and start exercising? What's the real reason? I truly hope it's for you. You have to do it for you and only you.

When the WHY gets stronger the HOW gets easier.

You see if you're just doing this to impress someone or make someone else happy then you're thinking about the wrong thing. You can't always make everyone happy. Start by making yourself happy because you deserve to be happy.

Life, Liberty and Pursuit of Happiness.

It has to be <u>for you</u> and <u>only you</u> to be long lasting and that's the real reason behind the curtain. If you're constantly trying to make others happy you'll never be happy. Those are called the facts.

Once you understand the WHY then the rest just falls into place. The WHY is more important than the HOW. Why you're doing something is 80% of the work. How to do something is 20%.

Don't get me wrong I'm here to guide you and help you lay out a blueprint to follow that will allow you to become successful with living healthy. So without further delay let's get started!

PART I: Identifying and Eliminating the Past
****

CHAPTER 1
An Exceptional Life Begins With Your Personal Philosophy

In physics it's said "A body in motion tends to stay in motion." This especially holds true when we're speaking of exercising and living healthy.

Many people have lots of "shoulds" in their lives. They should do this or they should do that. They basically should all over themselves! Should, could and would are not strong words. Or how about should, could or won't?

Should means you're careless. Won't probably means you're stubborn.

When is a good time to start something new? When the moment strikes you. When the idea hits you then capture it. If you want to start looking better, feeling better and living healthy it all starts now.

Never leave the site of a new goal without first doing something towards its achievement. Don't be casual about getting things, especially your health. Remember casualness leads to casualties.

FACT: A sedentary person loses a pound of muscle each year.

The formula for success:
A few simple disciplines practiced daily.

After today you can be a different person if you'll be willing to make these adjustments. You don't have to continue on the path you're on. The choice to take a different path starts with your thinking process.

Starting a new process doesn't need to require large amounts of action and connectivity even though those are the best type. Start with a small jog outside or a walk around the block but Just DO something!

What if I told you an apple a day keeps the doctor away? Would you eat the apple? Maybe. So you say I didn't have one yesterday and I'm fine but you got to be smarter than that. Just because yesterday nothing happened to you doesn't mean it won't hit you tomorrow.

So make a decision now to set your alarm clock a few minutes earlier and when it goes off GET UP! Don't just lie there and do nothing. Remember it only takes 3 weeks to develop a new habit. They say if you exercise for 6 months straight that you'll do it the rest of your life. Why? Because it becomes addictive. Once something becomes addicting you can't stop because there's always this urge to want more and do more. And that's where we're headed my friend.

Remember this,
"**If you keep doing what you're doing, you'll keep getting what you're getting**".

Ten years will pass regardless of what you decide to do with your health. The question is where will you be ten years from now?

You don't want to be that person when your older that has regrets. Regrets on what if you would've done this or what would life had been like if you would've made that one small change.

In the Navy we would change course just ever so slightly which didn't seem like a big deal. But guess what within just one day our destination changed dramatically and it all stemmed from one tiny change in our course.

Have you ever wondered what got you where you're at today? I was once asked who sold me on the plan I'm currently using. And I thought to myself what a fabulous question. Where did I get my current plan?

Do a little research and see what the main culprit behind so many health problems are. Can you guess?

OVERWEIGHT

Being overweight is related to diabetes, stroke, arthritis, breathing problems, depression, heart issues including heart attacks, knee problems to include knee replacement, stress based on the hormone cortisol, and many other things.

Even daily activities such as mowing your lawn, tying your shoes or playing with your kids becomes hard to do. It affects everything! Did you know asthma is reversible? It sure is!

FACT: A pound of fat is equal to 3500 calories.

Currently 3 out of 5 people are overweight and 1 out of 4 are obese in America. Worldwide 1.2 billion people are overweight. In the 1800's people used to eat ½ pound of sugar a year. Nowadays people eat 180 pounds of sugar a year!

While we're still covering the basics there's one more thing worth mentioning. I've heard people complain and say they've inherited their current situation. But let me let you in on a secret. Although heredity influences physical activity, fitness status and health, most people can lead healthy or unhealthy lives regardless of their genetic makeup. Thus genetic background neither dooms a person to poor health nor guarantee a high fitness level.

Now and at this very moment make the decision to change. Your decision will shape your entire future and touch on everything in your life. Going to Chapter 2 puts you ahead of the 90% whom never make it past this point. Read on my friend.

PART II: The Key to a Healthy and Successful Life Begins Now!

****

CHAPTER 2
First Principle- Nutrition

Why nutrition first you ask? Based on research and objective evidence eating is roughly 70% of getting in shape and losing weight. Remember you are what you eat. Junk in and junk out. I'm not going to preach much on eating your veggies BUT I will make my case and you decide what's right and wrong.

FACT: 80% of diets fail

Eating healthy is also known

as your diet. Don't get scared when you hear diet. It just means what you put into your stomach. When I refer to your diet I'm not talking about eating lettuce and branches from your front yard tree. I'm talking about changing your eating habits forever.

The world will not end if you eat a pizza or have a soda here and there. You have to enjoy life and reward yourself sometimes. At the same time you must be serious about what you really want. This isn't eat a few good meals for a week and then go back to stuffing anything down your throat program.

What would happen if a smoker said "Well I'll quit smoking for a week and see what happens"? I'm guessing they'll never kick the habit.

The same goes for your eating habits. You have to start eating right and continue to eat right. There is no other alternative or shortcut. Shortcuts lead to downfalls eventually and increases errors. And never forget this is your life we're talking about. Is there anything more important?

People have always amazed me when asking me what they should eat. Well for starters stop eating what you're currently eating.

A rule of thumb is when shopping stay on the outer edge of the store. These are foods that have to be kept cold and for good reason. They're real foods!

Milk, eggs, vegetables, meats, fruits and other items should make up the majority of your meals. Drink plenty of water, especially when awaking, 30 minutes before meals and before going to bed.

FACT: Drinking <u>16 ounces of water</u> increases metabolic rate by 25% in next hour.

What are nutrients? Nutrients are a combination of vitamins, minerals, carbohydrates, proteins (which are made up of amino acids), fats and water. All of these are absorbable components of foods – and necessary for good health.

Nutrients are necessary for energy, food utilization, organ functioning and overall cell growth. So it's pretty important. I hope you're sold on this fact because the sale is for you.

In essence there are two main groups: Macro-nutrients and Micro-nutrients. Macro-nutrients are proteins, fats and carbohydrates. Micro-nutrients are vitamins and minerals. You have to combine these groups in order to get energy.

Many people believe you can take some vitamins or minerals and have energy but it simply doesn't work this way. Your body needs ALL of the macro <u>and</u> micro nutrients in order to sustain high levels of peak performance.

Vitamins are simply organic substances and are essential to the normal functioning of the body. It's impossible to sustain life without vitamins. If your body was a car vitamins would be the spark plugs. Minerals are inorganic substances also essential to normal functioning of the body.

DID YOU KNOW?

It is not possible to obtain all the nutrients needed in your daily food intake?

Vitamins do not work without minerals and minerals do not work without vitamins.

Proteins, fats and carbohydrates you get from food. Foods such as eggs, lean meats, vegetables, fruits and whole grain food types are what the body needs.

Stick to real foods such as these and steer clear of processed foods, high fructose corn syrup foods, high in unsaturated fat foods, partially hydrogenated oil and pretty much anything that tastes yummy.

There's a saying that goes like this: "If it tastes good then it's probably not good for you."

Ice cream, candy, cakes, bagels, soda and pretty much anything that falls into those types of categories.

Concerning partially hydrogenated oil foods, the FDA's ruling is if the food has less than 0.5% partially hydrogenated oil per serving the food can be labeled as containing 0%! Wow!

So the food can actually contain partially hydrogenated oil but still say zero %! This is reason enough to read some of the nutritional facts on the side from now on. Just don't go by what you read and see on the outside of the package.

Determining BMI (Body Mass Index)

BMI is a measure of weight in relation to height:

BMI = weight in pounds x 703/height (inches) squared

Classification of Overweight and Obesity by BMI
In adults:

Healthy weight		18.5-24.9
Overweight		25.0-29.9
Obesity	Class I	30.0-34.9
	Class II	35.0-39.9
	Class III	≥40.0

"Stay on your nutrition. The average age in America is 75-78 years old."
Let's change it!!

Suggested Age-Based Body Fat Percentage Standards for Adults

Men
Recommended Range
18-34 years	8-22 %
35-55	10-25 %
56 years and older	10-25 %

Women
18-34	20-35 %
35-55	23-38 %
56 years and older	25-38 %

Your brain accounts for 2% of your weight but uses 20% of your energy!

FACT: 35% more sex are had by men who exercise between 3-4 days/week

The hardest part for getting in tip top shape for most people is the eating part! Why? Well if you think about it your around food all the time. Right?

You eat at least 3 times per day and can add to that whenever you want. Right? So we'll agree that eating is most difficult when you decide to change and get serious with your fitness.

Now don't get me wrong, like I said before its ok to enjoy life once in a while and reward yourself. But at the same time we have to be smart and know that this is a life changing ordeal and we're not doing this for nothing.

Protein shakes are a quick and easy way to stay healthy. Protein shakes can be designed and created based on what you want in your body. Some things to add are: protein (protein powder or eggs), oatmeal (one minute oat meal is fine), honey, peanut butter (powder version is healthier), chai seeds, coconut oil and dairy products such as almond milk or regular milk.

Almond milk is becoming the rage over regular milk based on its make-up and origins. Best of all are that protein shakes are yummy!

There are two types of protein which people usually get confused about. There is whey and casein protein. The difference lies with how quickly digesting they are.

For instance whey protein is digested in the body fairly quickly while casein protein is digested more slowly. For the majority of the population whey protein is what you're looking for.

When I was more into bodybuilding I would use casein protein in the middle of the night around 2AM because I was afraid of losing my gains I worked so hard to get from the gym. If you're not preparing for Mr. or Mrs. Olympia then whey protein is fine.

Protein powder can be purchased almost anywhere. If you own a SAM's card they have good deals. Word of wise for frugal folks like myself are purchase these products from wholesalers such as SAMs or Amazon if you are a subscriber. In the end you will receive just as good protein powder and save some money which can go towards other items of interest such as super greens, vitamins, water (I keep 3 cases on hand always) and other healthy things you will be needing.

Smoothies are an excellent source of nutrition and an easy way to maintain and stay on track. Not only are smoothies healthy but they taste delicious. Who says eating healthy doesn't taste good? The neat thing with smoothies is that you can design them anyway you want.

One important note here is try and ALWAYS use <u>vegetables</u> AND <u>fruit</u> when making you're smoothies. Make no mistake both are needed and required to achieve optimum health. With vegetables utilize different colors such as green, red, purple, orange and any other colors. The reasoning is behind phytonutrients which are chemical compounds that occur naturally in plants.

In plants phytonutrients protect the plant from UV rays or in others it protects from pest insecticides. When you consume these plants you will also derive health-promoting properties including antioxidant, anti-inflammatory, and liver-health-promoting activities.

Super greens are the rage and for good reasoning! They alkalize and energize! I wake up and drink a bottle of water every morning and then have my super greens drink afterwards before going to work. I usually mix mine with orange juice or pomegranate juice for flavor and additional nutrients.

Drinking water upon waking up starts your metabolism and after sleeping all night your body needs it!

By the way perform a body detox at least once per year. This cleanses your body and well worth it! I've always told my clients that there's no reason in purchasing a bunch of nutritional foods if your body is clogged up and unable to absorb them. I've never understood why most people don't detox.

While we're on this subject many people often wonder how much weight is idea for losing on a daily or weekly basis. The research indicates roughly 1-2 pounds per week is idea and safe.

One person that will not lie to you about your weight loss is the mirror. The mirror never lies.

The scale can be deceiving because let's say you lose a pound of fat but gain a pound of muscle then the scale says you haven't moved any. But in actuality you've done extremely well! Yes use the scale but just beware of this situation because it happens more often than not.

Another point to remember is that the first few days you may not see dramatic changes in your weight. Relax and do not think it's over before the journey begins. Just think how long it's been that you have been treating your body this way?

Some people will eat whatever for years and then think dropping 50 pounds overnight is going to happen. Folks if it was that easy America wouldn't have an overweight problem.

The first couple of lost pounds takes a few days. I use the analogy of starting a lawnmower. You give it a pull and then another pull. Then around the third or fourth pull BINGO!

So give your body some time and the weight will start to come off. Just believe in yourself and be consistent. Once the first pound leaves your body the next pound leaves. A domino effect begins and you'll never turn back my friend. A fire will ignite inside you and an addiction will take over.

Investing in yourself is the BEST thing you could ever do.

CHAPTER 3
Second Principle - Exercise

So far everything we've covered relates to your mental capacity and using your noggin on what to eat. Many people at this point turn the exercise part into building a new Death Star!

I've seen people almost write a book on their goals, pictures, plan of attack and so much more before even doing one sit-up! The goal here is to just get started!

My point is you don't need an engineering schematic with a 50 year blueprint to start out. Yes you want a plan and that's what this book entails. At this point we're discussing the exercise portion which will include either using weights or machines.

I prefer weights with a mix of machines. For the record men

usually utilize free weights while women like machines mostly. Maybe it's because when women look over at the free weight area there's 1.2 million men squeezed into that area all huffing and puffing!

Never let this be your deciding factor. The fact is you should mix it up as I do with free weights and machines to get the most from your workouts and it is the most effective way to truly reach your fitness goals. Also there's only so much you can do with free weights and that's where utilizing machines come to the rescue!

This book isn't covering how to utilize free weights or

machines. If you require assistance in that area I recommend using a friend that already works out or get a personal trainer. For the most part you can watch others and get a pretty good idea on how to use the weights and which part of the body is being worked out. Plus the machines have pictures depicting what body part is worked out.

Once we get older the machines are easier on the body and that's usually why you see elders utilizing machines.

I don't know where you're at concerning your health but I'm going to give you a blueprint on getting healthier and maintaining this level of fitness.

First thing you need to do is rid yourself of any bad habits such as smoking, excessive drinking or even drugs if you're that person. Those are called land mines and you should definitely stay away from them.

Maintaining a healthy body consists of three main parts.

- Eating healthy
- Exercising
- Proper rest

We've covered eating healthy and now its exercise time. I've read the average person has not stepped foot in a gym since graduating school!

Yikes! So we have some work ahead of us.

I'm going to break down the 3 key elements to maintaining a healthy body and in order of importance.

1. Cardiovascular Fitness
2. Strength
3. Flexibility

Is that what you were expecting? Probably not but when I became a certified personal trainer this is exactly what's being taught in the textbooks. Your cardio is number one based on keeping a healthy heart which works non-stop day in and day out.

To illustrate my example if you average 80 heart beats per minute that's 4,800 times per hour! Which is 115,000 per day and over 42 million times per year. If you reach 80 years old that's 3.3 billion heart beats!

So cardio is number one in maintaining your health. This includes walking, running, bicycle riding, swimming, rowing machines, elliptical machines, and any aerobic type activity such as Zumba or body pump classes. Even dancing is cardio and last but not least making love. Do that before going to the gym!

CARDIOVASCULAR FITNESS

If you're not an early bird like some folks then doing cardio after work is the only other option. But I'll tell you a secret if you decide to cardio in the morning you not only get it out of the way for the day but you crank up your metabolism! Great way to start any day off. It will literally increase your productivity throughout the day.

When you cardio you want to maintain about a 7 on the rector scale of 1-10 with 10 being the toughest. You're not trying to kill yourself, especially in the beginning.

You do want to get out of your comfort zone and sweat a little. My rule of thumb is if you didn't sweat then you're not getting out of your comfort zone which means you're really not doing much. Staying around a level 7 will ensure you not only sweat but you're not going overboard either.

FACT: 65% of women and men tone up for abs more than any other body part.

Some people when starting out will overdo things and then end up quitting which defeats the entire purpose. So your goal isn't to overdo it. It's to get started and enjoy the process.

Guess what will help engage you and help you enjoy the cardio process?

<u>Music</u>!

That's right put on those headphones and press play on your favorite playlist. Music will motivate you like no other and definitely assist you with getting through your cardio.

Some people after a period of time will listen to educational material instead of music. In that way you better manage your time! Maybe do this during your cool-down when you're finished exercising.

Twenty to thirty minutes at least 4 times per week for cardio. Actually 5 would be best since this will strengthen your heart and assist with toning up the body!

STRENGTH

Next is strength training and why is working muscles important? Did you know that muscle keeps your bone mineral density strong and gives you that ability to do everything you do from picking up objects to getting out of bed?

Another thing muscle does is that it increases your metabolism. Research shows that for every pound of new muscle you add your metabolism increases by burning an extra 30-40 calories an hour! The gift that keeps giving!

Again the object here isn't to break bones. It's to increase your strength and do it safely. Safety being the key here.

FACT: For every pound lost roughly 80% will be fat consistent with regular exercise

Again I recommend utilizing free weights and machines as a mixture. The different areas of the body are legs, both sides of arms, back, chest and shoulders.

An hour is an average amount of time for a workout consisting of resistance training and cardio.

Many folks skip leg day but don't you do that. The main reason besides having chicken legs is because when working legs it kicks up the most testosterone in the body.

Legs are the largest muscle group and helps the entire body grow as a whole. Legs are also considered compound movements. All this means is you get more work done in a shorter period of time.

To be honest if I was faced with being able to only work one single body part then it would definitely be legs. Legs are that important.

Ladies do not fear the word testosterone because we all have this hormone. The same goes for men having estrogen.

Many women think they will look like men of they work out too much. Trust me the women in the magazines work out "TONS" and it takes a long time to get that bulky. So don't worry.

Back to working legs. I usually mix shoulders in with legs. Legs don't take that long and it's a good mixture since your shoulders are fresh. Remember most of the time you work the larger muscle group first when you're at your highest energy level. Leg muscles take a lot of energy and are large muscles so hit them first whenever doing with another muscle group.

I'll usually work chest with biceps (part of arm everyone flexes to show off). Always work the largest muscle first so in this case it's definitely the chest. Also by working these two together you create a push and pull workout.

What do I mean? Chest is a pushing exercise and that's why we call them pushups. Biceps is a pulling exercise. So in essence you're working a large muscle group and a small group which is a good combination.

Lastly you have back and triceps. Again one large

muscle group with a small group. Back is pulling and triceps are a pushing movement so that's a good combination.

Remember to work the larger group first. In this case it's your back muscle and then your triceps.

After a while you will definitely know how to work out using weights and machines. At that point try mixing things up. Maybe instead of doing all chest and then biceps you can perform one chest exercise and then one bicep exercise. Back and forth until you have completed three sets per body part.

Since we're talking about weights and machines, now let's quickly go over sets versus repetitions.

Every muscle needs to be exhausted which just means it requires to be pushed to their limits. A rule of thumb over the years is to perform 3 different exercises per body part.

For each different exercise you will perform 3 sets. Usually a set consists of 10-12 repetitions. So for chest you do 3 different exercises. Let's assume you do the bench press. You will do the bench press three different times and each time you will push for 10-12 repetitions. That completes one exercise and now you still have two exercises left.

This goes for each body part. Since body parts are different your exercises performed for those different body parts will also be different. Meaning you can't work your biceps doing flat bench because flat bench is for chest.

Let's not forget the Holy Grail...ABDOMINALS!! Also referred to as abs. These guys are similar to distant cousins. You never see them but you know they're there!

Well the good news is that these are pretty tough muscles which means you can work them 2-3 times per week. Don't leave out the Swiss ball either. Your abs work over 50% harder when using Swiss ball versus the bench or floor!

I placed abs last since the best comes last. My point is do your ab training when your finished working out. It's easier and you'll work your abs harder because you're in a heightened state.

While we're talking strength let's see what the difference is between strength and endurance. Are they the same? Not at all but they're related.

Strength is just that. How much weight can a specific muscle group pick up or push

one time. While endurance relates to **how many times** can a certain amount of weight be picked up or pushed.

Say you know a friend that can bench press 315 for a one time rep max. Your other friend can bench press 225 but for 35 repetitions. Let me ask you a question. Can the friend that benches 315 pounds do more reps at 225 pounds than your other friend? Maybe. But in some cases your friend cannot.

At the same time your friend benching 225 pounds for 35 repetitions might not be able to bench 315 pounds either.

So my point is strength is how much weight at one time a person can lift versus how much weight can be lifted numerous times. Over and over.

Your muscle is made up of slow twitch and fast twitch fibers. The simplest way to ensure you work both types of fibers is to go heavy AND light. One week push yourself some with a little weight. On another week go lighter but bump up your repetitions. This simple technique will ensure you are maximizing your workouts and create what's called a shocking principle for your body.

FACT: The average male can do 35 sit-ups in 60 seconds

FLEXIBILITY

The third component of being healthy and creating fitness is flexibility. Flexibility relates to the ability to bend without breaking.

When exercising you will need to bend and flex in order to do what's necessary to get in shape or maintain your fitness. Having functional range of motion at all joints of the musculoskeletal system is desirable to ensure efficient body movement.

Ever notice when a cat awakens that they immediately stretch. Military stretches every morning prior to conducting physical fitness. Stretching is critical.

Stretching before AND after exercising is best. I've read that stretching before is more a mental thing but I've always done it and suggest you do it too. Stretching afterwards is really good because the muscles are warmed up and stretch easier.

Do not do hard core stretching before working out! I've seen people walk into the gym and go crazy on their stretching as if they were trying to resemble Gumby! This can cause you an injury so take it easy when stretching prior to working out. Remember you're just warming up.

Stretching will keep you limber and increases skeletal structure. Yoga is an excellent form of stretching. Again make it a point to stretch before AND after exercising. Around 5-10 minutes each time is good enough.

Recap Time

Cardio at least 4 times a week but we're really looking for 5 times.

With strength training we're looking for every body part being hit once a week. Remember to perform 3 different exercises for each muscle group. And do 3 sets per exercise which is the minimum. This will give you the best results.

Before and after cardio or strength training we will be stretching. Do not forget to stretch! When you stretch after you've worked out it not only feels good but gives you a chance to cool down and is extremely good for the body.

Before leaving the gym I want to tell you to take advantage of any amenities. Many gyms have saunas, steam rooms, swimming pools, hot tubs, racquetball courts and more.

Utilize these other avenues at a minimum to see if you like

them. But more importantly to receive the benefits of them that you cannot get from just exercising. Plus you've already paid for these amenities so you might as well use them!

CHAPTER 4
Third Principle - Rest

Sleep plays a critical role in your physical health. Being well rested is the analogy of charging up a battery.

To make things worse if you exercise and workout while being tired you can reverse your gains and actually go backwards with your health! Referred to as atrophy which is a reduction in muscle fiber.

Believe it or not some beginners fall into this atrophy category and when gains or weight loss are not immediately evident they quit and never not realize WHY they were not successful.

Knowledge is power so remember this when you're up late at night trying to finish a movie or just awake.

SLEEP, LEARNING, and MEMORY

It may not be surprising that it is more difficult to take in new information following a night of insufficient or troubled sleep. What's more surprising is that it is just as significant to get a good night's sleep after learning something new in order to process and remember the information that has been learned.

Research suggests that sleep supports learning and memory in two distinctive ways.

First, a tired person cannot focus attention optimally and therefore cannot learn proficiently.

Second, sleep itself has a role in the partnership of memory, which is important for learning new information.

When cops speak to individuals about drinking and driving they tell people that not sleeping for 24 hours is similar to blowing 0.08 on the blood alcohol content analyzer! Basically no sleep means your drunk! Not the best thing when we're pushing our bodies and working on changing our physiques.

Sleep is a necessary part of life and many of us scrape by with little as possible. Many well-known health personnel relate sleep as a pillar of optimal health.

Sleep regulates the production of most hormones meaning while your asleep the body produces many important hormones. Human growth hormone is produced when in deep sleep coming from your pituitary glands.

The body generates less of this hormone as we age.

These hormones can make or break your ability to perform at high levels, prevent cancer and other diseases, and the much needed losing weight as well.

Some will turn to pharmaceutical pills which studies are showing that just a small amount during a year can increase your chances of death. Not to mention these pills only add a few minutes of sleep at best per night.

Some benefits of sleep if you're still not a believer:

✓ Healthier skin

- ✓ **Easier to control your emotions**
- ✓ **Decreases risk of diseases**
- ✓ **Keeps hormones in check**
- ✓ **Helps with weight loss**
- ✓ **More effective immune system**
- ✓ **Longevity**
- ✓ **Fewer errors and accidents**
- ✓ **And many more positives are associated with proper sleep.**

Studies reflect that more than 65% of Americans suffer from sleep loss.

Just a mere century ago people slept an average of 2-3 hours longer. So what happened?

Remember from Chapter 1 we talked about your inherited heredity has nothing to do with getting the body you've always desired. The same holds true with sleep.

I've heard others talk about having a certain gene that prevents them from good solid sleep. Many people bought into this gene theory. Well don't you fall for it!

Our genes do play a role but everything from your experiences growing up, your surroundings, and even your lifestyle have something to do with determining which genes our bodies turn to.

In essence your genes and DNA are the blueprint or schematic that the body utilizes. So as you go through life and do the different things and associate with whomever your body is using this to restructure your blueprint.

Huge studies are following these activities and the new field of science entitled epigenetics has emerged.

Just like we didn't know that lead in the air was cancerous or asbestos could eventually kill you the same goes for figuring more out about our genes. It's very interesting. Best part about it is we are not slaves to our genetics or genes.

The numbers are in and I can tell you unequivocally that less sleep affects everything you do. Especially working out! Utilize this strategy and ensure you are getting the optimum amount of sleep. Your body will thank you.

CHAPTER 5 - Ideas for Inspiration and Making Yourself a Little Bit Better

My philosophy has always been to improve yourself and do a little bit better every day. In addition to getting the body you've always desired and achieving this as the ultimate goal, some wonder what else they can do to improve upon themselves.

This chapter will shed some light in these areas as well as debunk some myths that you may have heard or even believe.

For instance you hear women say using free weights and getting too bulky is a man thing. At the same time you hear guys talk about getting a pedicure is for the ladies. Again if you believe those words then you're truly missing out on part of the good life my friend.

Some of these are ideas that can better yourself or maybe just for pleasure. Either way I believe them to be part of the "good life".

MEDITATION

The first item of interest is meditation. Yes meditation. Why meditation? Life is chaotic and we lose sight of where and what we want I believe. Rushing to get something done, shoveling down your food and tasting it later, not being happy with where you're at in life and on and on.

Our goal is to get in shape and live healthy correct? Well it's often said that the major reason for setting a goal is for what it makes of you to accomplish it. What it makes of you will always be far greater value than what you get.

So why not enjoy yourself as you grow and become a better person. Rome wasn't built overnight and enjoying the process as much as the destination is one of the keys to success. So let's start the enjoyment!

Meditation isn't some mysterious act that people high in the mountains perform. When I'm asked about meditation most people say "They started meditation but stopped". I also hear "I would love to learn how to meditate".

So when it comes down to it these are some of the reasons why people don't meditate from what I've heard:

✓ It's way too complicated.
✓ It takes a lot of time.
✓ I'm not the spiritual type.
✓ I'm too old.
✓ I'm not good enough.
✓ I'm not the brainy type.
✓ I'm too young.

Then there are those that started meditating and stopped. The following are their reasons:

✓ Took too long.
✓ Wasn't the spiritual type.
✓ Didn't get anything from it.

I'm betting these are their rational thoughts. But this is just scratching the surface. Underneath and a little deeper I believe it boils down to 2 things.

- ✓ Mediation was confusing and hard.
- ✓ Trying to learn mediation and it actual took too long.

The second rational could hold some truth based on there being over 10,000 books on meditation out there! Mix the readings with what people have heard or been told and the next thing you know there's mass confusion. Confusion leads to fear which then becomes quitting.

The amount of time to actually meditate is 7 minutes! That's it! Who doesn't have 7 minutes to spare on a daily basis?

- That equates to 2 commercials while watching TV or to make a sandwich for yourself.
- Go to bed 7 minutes earlier or go to bed 7 minutes later if you perform at night.

So what is meditation? In short form and to keep it simple <u>meditation is allowing what is to be at that point in time.</u>

So for the next minute close your eyes and place your hands in your lap. Breathe in a deep breath and just listen. Hear the cars go by outside, and as alert as possible say to yourself.

Meditation is allowing life to be.
Meditation is allowing life to be.
Meditation is allowing life to be.

Do you feel something? What was it you felt? Did you know that meditation is good for you?

Over the past half century there have been numerous studies covering the effects of meditation. Some of the research shows that meditation can:

✓ Relieve stress
✓ Reduce anxiety

- ✓ **Loosen up internal organs**
- ✓ **Increase lung capacity**
- ✓ **Increase efficiency of breathing**
- ✓ **Lower chronic and acute pain**
- ✓ **Decrease blood pressure**

So let's keep in mind that in order to mediate we're not missing out on reading our trashy novels or sports magazines, we're not getting involved in a religious ordeal, we're definitely not avoiding the real world (actually the opposite is happening), you're not being hypnotized, and you don't have to be in total silence. The list goes on but these just aren't true.

Before getting any further something that can be counterproductive when meditating is continually opening your eyes to see the time. Now would be a perfect time to invest in a kitchen timer or egg timer. Their about $5 and well worth it.

You've probably seen people sitting with their legs crossed on huge fluffy pillows. Well this isn't necessary. Sitting upright in a chair with your hands on your lap and your posture straight but rested is perfect. Eyes closed and breathing with your own rhythm. Find your breathing.

Meaning you may breathe better from down below versus up top by your throat.

Don't skip this section because it sets the pace for everything.

Mediation is letting your thoughts just flow from one to another. Experience whatever enters your mind and go with the flow. I've imagined bicycle riding and then going on liberty call while visiting Africa while in Navy and then going out to an awesome dinner with my wife! Now how does all of this mix and have to do with one another. I have no idea.

Meditation allows you to be free and let be. Thoughts will come and go. One point here is to meditate on your breathe. Meaning watch you're breathing and staying on mark.

I thought this would be an easy task and when I first tried to watch and be conscious of my breathing. I found myself thinking about the Iraq war I was part of and then I was competing in a bicycle contest and then I remembered the guy cutting me off while driving the day before!

So when you're meditating watch your breathing, if you stray off course then notice it and gently return to your breathing.

In the world of meditation there's what's called "catching and releasing".

Similar to fishing. This comes in handy for those thoughts that derail your thought process like the guy that cut me off while driving and my entire thought process from there is finding an Army to locate this guy and start World War III!

In essence you're just realizing that you're off path and come back to noticing you breathing. Your breathing pattern will allow you to remain on track and focused.

So let's begin:

- Notice where in your body that you're most conscious of the feeling of breathing.

- **Maintain direction to this area of your body, secure point.**

- **Observe your breathing and notice your normal breathing pattern.**

- **Remember to let in and try not to learn anything here. Just let in and let be.**

- **Straying off. Notice and return to your secure point.**

- **Perform a full breath in and out. Stay on mark.**

- **Getting irritated. Come back to breathing and recognize it.**

- How are we doing on breathing?

- Continue this until the timer sounds.

- Congratulations you have just completed meditation!

The reality is that your minds job is to think – 24 hours a day! It's not going to stop because you want to meditate for 7 minutes.

When you stop trying to stop your thoughts, you begin to surpass them. *The beauty is this can lead you to peace and serenity that you probably only thought you could achieve when you stopped thinking!*

Last but not least never forget you're A, B, C's. Always Be Calm. This statement alone is worth many lessons learned in life by itself. This "Always Be Calm" is not only for meditation but life itself.

MASSAGES

I've often wondered why more people do not get massages. It's always fascinated me because massages feel so good. So why aren't more people getting them? Time, money, not a touchy type person, they don't do anything, and so on might be some of the answers based on interviewing people and questions I've asked.

The real deal is that massages are an excellent source of stress relief and can assist with healing of the body naturally.

Below are some of the benefits from massages:

Even if you don't have a specific health issue, massage therapy can provide many benefits, such as:

- ✓ Increased circulation
- ✓ Digestive disorders
- ✓ Stimulation of the lymph system, the body's natural defense against toxic invaders

- ✓ Release of endorphins, the body's natural painkiller
- ✓ Sports injuries
- ✓ Improved range of motion and decreased discomfort associated with lower back pain
- ✓ Relaxation of injured and overused muscles
- ✓ Reduced muscle spasms and cramping
- ✓ Increased joint flexibility
- ✓ Help recover from strenuous workouts
- ✓ Pain relief from headaches
- ✓ Reduce post-operative adhesions and edema, as well as reduced scar tissue

Since this is a book on health and fitness I'll let you in on a secret amongst professional bodybuilders. They all receive massages. Usually deep tissue massages based on trying to appear larger by separation between muscle and bone. Plus it feels great!

Regular monthly massages provides therapeutic relief to people of all ages and all walks of life, from the competitive athlete to the home kitchen chef to the health physics instructor person.

Here's why: Massage offers a non-invasive, drug free and humanistic approach to wellness based on the body's natural ability to heal itself.

Massages are no longer available only through luxury spas and upscale health clubs. Today, massage therapy is offered in businesses, clinics, hospitals and even airports. If you've never tried massage, learn about its possible health benefits and what to expect during a massage therapy session.

Types of Massages:

- **Swedish Massage - This is a gentle form of massage that uses long strokes, kneading, deep circular movements, vibration and tapping to help relax and energize you.**

- **Deep Massage - This massage technique uses slower, more-forceful strokes to target the deeper layers of muscle and connective tissue, commonly to help with muscle damage from injuries.**
- **Sports Massage - This is similar to Swedish massage, but it's geared toward people involved in sport activities to help prevent or treat injuries.**
- **Trigger Point Massage - This massage focuses on areas of tight muscle fibers that can form in your muscles after injuries or overuse.**

Plus there are other services offered that feel just as good

and are good for the body. Below I've listed some of the more utilized ones.

- ✓ **Body Scrub - Helps remove dead skin and expose younger looking supple skin. Body Scrubs at helps to rejuvenate the skin by exposing the smoother and supple layer of skin after removal of the dead skin layer**

- ✓ **Body Wraps - A 'mask' is applied all over the body before being wrapped in a thermal blanket, allowing the body's heat to activate the absorption of the natural ingredients.**

- ✓ **Foot Scrubs - Salt dehydrates skin and that's why foot scrub's feature sugar. Its naturally hydrating properties soothe and smooth for a more refreshing experience which feels great!**

- ✓ **Hot Stone Message - Hot stone massage therapy melts away tension, eases muscle stiffness and increases circulation and metabolism.**

There are other services out there that include more but this should give a picture. If you have never received a massage I deplore you to

schedule one and see for yourself. They truly are overlooked by people that need them.

PEDICURES

Well you're saying this guy has to be joking. The furthest thing from the truth my friend. If your one of those men that believe this is a woman thing then you're definitely missing out on the "good life".

The ladies know what I'm talking about. Some probably wish their better halves would try it. Not only are pedicures great for the feet but will give you more time with your spouse if you want to double date on this.

Let's face it your feet are probably the most used body part. From the minute you awake you're on those dogs and that's not even including if you run or do any vigorous exercising.

The average person takes 8,000 to 10,000 steps a day, which adds up to about 115,000 miles over a lifetime! All this wear and tear on your feet can be harmful if they are not maintained properly.

Again just like massages if you've never received a pedicure then today is your day. Nowadays they serve adult beverages while you're sitting in a massage chair!

Where in the world can you go, be served a drink, receiving a body massage and have the most overworked part of your body fixed? Trust me you'll wonder why you never did it after your first visit.

Here are some benefits of a pedicure:

- ✓ Receiving a regular pedicure can help the pedicurist detect early marks of corns, bunions and fungal infections.

- ✓ Clipping, cutting and cleaning of the toe nails prevents them from inward growth and causing infection.

- ✓ A pedicure includes soaks in warm water and massages with oils and lotions that help preserve the moisture and truth of your feet. Moisturized feet are less likely to get blisters, crakes or other foot problems.

- ✓ The removal of the dead skin on your feet, especially on the heel, inspires new cell growth which creates smoother and good-looking feet.

- ✓ The most enjoyable part of the pedicure is the massage. That's right another massage!

Massaging helps promotes circulation and helps relieve tension in the calves and feet. Increase in blood passage can reduce pain and help dispense heat throughout your body.

✓ Pedicure can be very relaxing. It helps you relieve stress and can be therapeutic.

As I was saying earlier feet receive little to no care. The face and hands seem to get all the attention. Not to mention healthy feet lead to a better life overall. You need your feet so start taking better care of them.

****

CHAPTER 6 -Rules of Engagement

1. No pain - no gain. Pain from soreness is ok. Pain from injuries isn't. Know the difference and understand when your body is telling you to stop.

2. When your there be there. Don't waste your time because you can't get it back. <u>Make use of your time and get results</u>. Too many people socialize and hang out instead of getting something accomplished. It's ok to talk while you're working out but don't turn it into a social event.

3. *Use gym etiquette*. Don't stand in front of the dumb bell rack while using them, get an idea of who's using what before taking over a piece of equipment, wipe off equipment when your done and overall bring a great attitude.

4. Bring what's known as the essentials. Small towel, <u>water</u>, knee wraps, <u>music</u> and your written routine if needed. More serious folks who are power lifting or CrossFit may have an entire bag with them. If you're going to utilize showers and such then definitely bring shower shoes.

5. Know what time of the day is best for you. Everyone is

different. Mine is between 9am-1pm. I've tried squatting 400 lbs. at 5:30am and definitely not for me.

6. Having a workout partner is an excellent idea. I've worked out with up to 2 more individuals but you have to keep moving. Two people is perfect. Plus they can spot you in times when you're moving up in weight. *Rule of thumb is to work out with someone stronger than you*. This way they push you. The other way and you're pushing them which helps them grow faster and not you.

7. Its best to eat a couple hours prior to working out. Your body <u>requires energy</u>

and not a bunch of crap from the local so called nutrition store. People buy all this crazy stuff when what's really needed is either a protein shake or something healthy. So save your money.

8. Take some time and develop your fitness goals. *You can't manage what you can't measure*. Take a picture of yourself and get your exact weight before you begin your journey to success. This enables you to track your progress. Later on these numbers come in handy when figuring out how far you've come. The mirror never lies so use it!

10. Do what <u>feels right</u> to you. There will inevitably be days when you truly aren't in the right mind or mood to work out. We all have these days. In these situations just chill and relax. Call it your cheat day. I've discovered that pushing through and still working out isn't sometimes the best.

11. Once in a while take a week off. And by doing so I don't mean on a monthly basis! Yes you read that right. *The body is unique and deserves a break from time to time.* It will sort of recalibrate the body because it's so use to exercising and now it can in a way start over. Except this time in

much better shape.

12. If you hire a personal trainer ensure you follow their instructions. Inevitably they will assign you homework. Make sure you do this because it's all part of your plan to reaching your fitness goals. I've had clients in the past who would not do their homework and then want to blame me when their numbers didn't drop fast enough. Again it goes back to not wasting your time or money. *Time is more important because you can't get it back but you can make more money*. Days are expensive.

13. <u>You grow outside the gym.</u> But you break down the

body when you're in the gym. Again ensure you get serious and get to work while you're in the gym.

14. Last but not least don't over-do it. <u>Pick up the weights that you're body allows you to pick up.</u> A rule of thumb is find out what you can lift/pull at 12 repetitions and then increase the weight but lower your reps for the next set.

15. Once in awhile buy a new exercise outfit or new pair of shoes. Reward your hard work. It feels good to wear something new into the gym.

16. After working out for 6 months you'll do it the rest of your life. Exercising is that

addicting.

17. There's no such thing as failures. There are only results. You might not always like the results but that's what they are and you can change them.

CHAPTER 7 – Crossing Over and Applying Principles to Change Your Life Forever

At this point I'm sure you're full of excitement and ideas. These are the feelings you should be having and with it comes attitude that you can do it.

This is the time you need to get up and make the change

you've always only thought about up until now.

I can tell you from my own experiences that when you get bit by the health bug you'll definitely know it! You'll be thinking about exercising at work, on the way to work and home, before going to sleep and just about all the time because you have now found a new hobby but honestly this is way more than a hobby.

This is something that will not only change your body and give you the body you've always desired but will touch on EVERYTHING you do in life.

- You'll notice you sleep better because now

you're really physically tired and will help you sleep.
- Your daily activities become easier such as mowing the lawn or tying you're shoes.
- Your memory improves which helps with work and at home life.
- Your energy levels increase and gives you the ability to do more in the same amount of time.
- Lastly your stress disappears. <u>Remember stress ALWAYS leads to fear.</u> Become grateful for your new profound activities and fear will cease to exist. Whenever you're grateful fear disappears.

It's funny because so many people are under stress. I don't care where you live there's some sort of stress your feeling on a daily basis. And if you follow stress it always leads to fear.

The sad thing is that people that are stressed will not exercise and that's the one thing that will alleviate and get rid of their stress! Do you believe me? I hope so because the sales for you like I said.

Once you really get serious and start your workout routine you will notice all of these wonderful benefits I've explained here.

Living a healthy life touches on anything and everything you do. Trust me you do not want to retire and not be able to enjoy yourself because you didn't take better care of yourself.

"Start now. A body in motion tends to stay in motion."

I wish you the very best and really hope you put this information to good use.

During reading my eBook you should have had that mental conversation with yourself about making changes and deciding that now is the best time! I challenge you to do something different at this very moment. Don't wait for the urge to go away and <u>do</u>

not put off any longer. It's been long enough.

People can achieve anything and that definitely includes you. You can at this moment decide to start getting in better shape, lose unwanted weight, quit smoking and most of all getting started and changing your life forever!

Please email me at yourfreebook@mattaubert.com and share with me your successes concerning your health and fitness goals once you've achieved them or if you have questions concerning health and fitness.

FREE DOWNLOAD

**Sign up for the author's New Releases
mailing list and get a free copy of the
latest Turning Bad Habits into Success.**

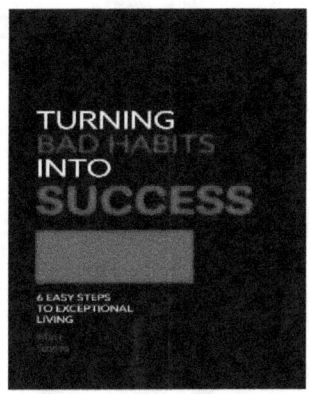

Click here to get started:
www.StartLiving.com

**Again thank you for reading.
Please write a review which
follows on the next page and
let me know what my book
has done for you. Will you
make the necessary changes
based on what I have
provided you? Are there any**

other items of interest I can help you with?

I wish you the very best and really hope you put this information to good use.

www.ingramcontent.com/pod-product-compliance
Lightning Source LLC
Chambersburg PA
CBHW070152290526
45789CB00002B/739